Stork's Journey

Stork's Journey

A Guide for Intended Parents considering Gestational Surrogacy sans Agency

M. L. Sejour

ISBN-13: 9781523343638
ISBN-10: 152334363X

Now to Him who is able to do Immeasurably more than all I can ask or imagine…

For Ellie – You are Joy Unspeakable

To Ashley and many women who give couples hope….you are the ray of sunshine after the storm.

For my Love - DY: We did it! She is absolutely beautiful.

Contents

CHAPTER 1

This Is Really Happening!

IT TOOK MANY months for us to come to terms with the idea that gestational surrogacy was the only remaining viable option for my husband and me to have a child who would be genetically related to us. After a few years of multiple surgeries—removing uterine fibroids; removing my left ovary due to an ovarian cyst; removing an ovarian abscess from my right ovary due to infection post an egg retrieval procedure; and due to blocked fallopian tubes from my first myomectomy—I was very grateful for modern medicine and the option of gestational surrogacy. Unlike some couples who struggle with unexplained infertility, I had the mixed blessing of knowing the medically diagnosed reasons why it was nearly impossible for me to conceive and carry a child. Knowing that it was highly risky for me to try to carry a child, I began to look into options that would enable my husband and me to have a child of our own. I discovered the option of gestational surrogacy—the process by which a surrogate would be implanted, through IVF, with an embryo created from my egg and my husband's sperm.

It took me several months off and on during 2014 to research the surrogacy process and better understand the role of the surrogacy agency. It seemed like an involved, costly, and overwhelming process. For a period of time, I allowed the cost and complexity to discourage me. I almost resigned myself to having a childless household. This is fine for some, but I knew in my heart of hearts that I wanted children. I spent months seeking God's guidance, writing petition prayers, finding and studying biblical scriptures related to being barren or not having children, and educating myself about all the options I could employ to become a mother. Both my heart (my faith and will) and my head (my intellect) were engaged, so everything aligned.

I contacted a few surrogacy agencies, but I grew disillusioned with the process because there seemed to be such a long wait to be matched with a surrogate. There was already a lengthy waiting list for surrogates in our state, and surrogates from other surrogate-friendly states were in high demand. I was growing anxious because I did not know how long our frozen embryos would remain viable. At that point, it was coming up on one full year from the time when the embryos had been created. Everything I had heard told me I should not wait any longer if we wanted a real chance to have our own children. Around that time, I learned there were independent avenues for surrogacy. This independent avenue meant something significant. If I did not have a friend or relative who could be a surrogate and if I did not want to work through a surrogacy agency, there was a virtual place—a place online—where I could find a surrogate who would be the best match for my baby and me.

My decision not to work through an agency was purely financial. Other individuals might decide against working with agencies for financial, time-related, or personal reasons. I was determined to pay for surrogacy without having to go into debt. After all, surrogacy can be quite costly. Between my savings and incoming bonus at the time, I made it happen. If I had signed on with a surrogacy agency, I would have had to pay $5,000 or more for an entity to screen and coordinate everything. Given my goal oriented nature and knowing that I was up for the challenge, I decided to take on the task myself. That's not to say I knew I would do a better job than a surrogacy agency, but with tight financial resources, it was worth an attempt. I'm sure there are wonderful and effective surrogacy agencies making differences in the lives of intended parents (people who become the legal parents of a child born through surrogacy) everywhere. The surrogacy agencies are there to guide parents through the process and, in most cases, will take on the chief coordination role for their clients. I have nothing bad to say about any surrogacy agency, but I needed to find another way.

My discovery of the independent avenue was serendipitous. My husband had worked with someone several years ago who was a first time surrogate for a would be single mother. My husband was able to locate his former coworker, and that coworker was all too happy to provide the contact details for the past intended parent/single mom. I largely have my husband to thank for finding this path for us. That intended parent informed me about Surrogate Mothers Online LLC (Surromomsonline.com). She spent more than an hour educating me about the process and sharing her past experiences. Surromomsonline.com is a virtual meeting place for the surrogacy community. Intended parents can meet surrogates there and vice versa. After speaking with her, I decided to check out the website.

I began this process in the summer of 2014. Initially, I began by answering the ads of gestational surrogates. I answered at least twelve ads but received no follow-up responses. I grew disheartened. I wondered whether I had provided too much information or perhaps not the right kind of information. It was not entirely a surprise, though, because the past intended parent had warned me I might not hear back. Even so, when I received no replies, I temporarily suspended the pursuit. I regrouped, however, in the fall of 2014 after I learned that a very close friend was expecting a baby. Like most women who struggle to conceive, pregnancy announcements trigger mixed feelings. You are always happy for the woman or couple, but it's yet another dagger in your heart—a reminder of your own plight. This time around, I was optimistic, hopeful, and very encouraged I would be sharing my own great news in a few months. I decided to post an ad for my husband and me as intended parents. Our ad was short, but it addressed the pertinent elements. It read something like this:

> We are a loving married couple of five years (thirty-four and forty years old) looking for a gestational surrogate.
>
> • Stable marriage and relationship—the first and only marriage for both of us
> • No children from prior relationships or together

- Hardworking professionals
- Reside in the Midwest
- Drug-free individuals
- Three embryos (two girls and one boy), already genetically and gender tested
- I cannot carry due to medical reasons

We are ready to go!

Looking for an experienced gestational surrogate with insurance. We would like our surrogate to reside in the Midwest, but we would consider a GC (gestational carrier) residing elsewhere based on match and surrogacy laws. Our preference is to find someone prepared, experienced, and serious. You must have all recent physical, medical, and mental evaluations and tests completed.

Within one hour of posting my ad, I received inquiries from several potential surrogates (from all over the United States) via phone and e-mail. As I corresponded with them over two to three weeks, I learned so much about many things (e.g., state surrogacy laws, compensation, the milestones of the process, etc.). I found a few of the experienced surrogates very insightful, and they helped me better understand the process.

Ultimately, the gestational surrogate (also known as "gestational carrier" or "GC") I selected was a bit older than I would have wanted, but she had a proven track record. She was keen on keeping a healthy diet as well. Most importantly, while some surrogates with whom I had become acquainted seemed to be out to get rich, she was trying to find ways I could save money. I appreciated this immensely. She reassured me I could take an independent avenue without having to work through an agency or go into serious debt.

Even though my husband got me in touch with the past intended parent, it took my husband some time to accept the process. He wanted me to have had the experience of carrying our child. The fact there was going to be a third party involved (i.e., the gestational carrier) made him anxious and uncomfortable. He had concerns the carrier might want to keep our child. Our own psychological evaluation session (legally required) was helpful early on in getting him on board. The psychological evaluation was required based on the laws of the state where our surrogate lived and would give birth. In addition, the surrogate and her partner had to complete a psychological evaluation too. During our psychological evaluation session, the licensed psychologist validated my husband's feelings and reassured him it was OK to feel what he was feeling. After our session, I noticed a positive change in my husband. He was glad not to have felt judged because he had reservations about the process. My husband did not want to remain in contact with the gestational carrier after the birth of our child. He was grateful the carrier wanted to give us this gift, but he often would remind me she was being fairly compensated for the surrogacy service. He grew a little more comfortable with embarking on the journey as time went by, but I could tell with every passing month that the anticipation of the big day (when our daughter would be born) weighed on him. The psychologist allowed us to realize that this decision was no small feat and that we should take the necessary time to absorb all stages of the process.

Call it motherly instincts, but I was our lead cheerleader throughout the process. I cheerfully handled all the details between us and our surrogate's family, as well as arranged the hospital plans. My husband was supportive, but he had limited interaction and communication with the surrogate and her family. I knew my husband would be supportive in other ways while getting ready for the birth of our child. I would not describe my husband as the touchy-feely type. He is more of a man's man. His priorities were making sure our daughter had a safe and comfortable home to come to and making sure we were building an adequate financial nest for the big life changes coming. From month to month, he would check in with me on the surrogacy payments and milestones to see how things were progressing. While I was the face to the surrogate, my husband was my sounding board and well of encouragement. He was an ear on the days I grew frustrated with a few hiccups along our journey.

You don't have to be perfect for the surrogacy process to be success-
ful. It is best, however, to have a healthy and loving marriage in which
both partners are committed to each other, their marriage, and raising
the child they are bringing into the world within that marriage. You
should discuss all your thoughts and feelings throughout the process—
good and bad. Be honest with one another. Know and discuss what roles
you will play. This is surrogacy, after all. While surrogacy is growing in
popularity for couples struggling with infertility, it is a very different
and somewhat unconventional way for parents to bring children into
the world. Don't minimize the process or experience. Affirm this is the
decision you made, and don't look back.

Allow yourself to feel and think the full range of emotions and
thoughts. For example, there were days early in the process when I could
not understand why my surrogate wanted more interaction and communication than I was allowing myself to provide. Over time, the bond
we developed came naturally. Before it did though, I'm sure she thought
I was too businesslike and private, and I felt she was wanted more from
me emotionally than what I was prepared to give. Since my daughter
was born, I cannot recall a time when the bumps along the surrogacy
process surfaced again in my thoughts. These moments are no longer
important, and they have no bearing on our lives today. However, in the
midst of these bumps, I shed tears and confronted my own vulnerability.

When my surrogate was twenty-seven weeks along, she had a regular
doctor's appointment. Of course, I joined the appointment via Skype.
The appointment seemed noneventful, and things with my daughter
were fine. Little did I know the twenty-four hours following the appointment would be stressful. My surrogate called me back thirty minutes
after the appointment and indicated she had been experiencing tightness in her lower abdomen during the standard ultrasound, but she had
been concerned about saying anything for fear she would cause unnec-
essary alarm. She had engaged in sexual intercourse the night before
the doctor appointment, which might have caused the fetal fibronectin
screen (a test to check if the amniotic sac remains "glued" to the lining
of the uterus) to yield a positive result. This combination led to what

seemed a perfect storm of complete panic. The symptom of abdomen tightness and the positive fetal fibronectin results were all signs that pointed to preterm labor. In the event my surrogate was going through preterm labor, she was given a shot of steroids to help expedite the development of my daughter's lungs.

I was absolutely humbled and nearly devastated that my surrogate could be going through preterm labor and that my daughter would have to be born nearly 3 months early. Being someone who exercises control in the sphere of my life and makes sure things are always buttoned up, I was floored I could not control this circumstance. All I could do was trust my God and provide as such moral support to my surrogate as possible. I was very grateful my husband kept his cool and was the voice of reason and encouragement to my surrogate and me. This hiccup could have happened to anyone—regardless of whether choosing the indie route or taking the journey via a surrogacy agency. This anecdote only reflects the fragility of conception and real obstacles encountered by expecting parents.

Once you have started the surrogacy process or have decided to take that path, it's up to you to decide how much information to disclose to family and friends. One piece of advice I got before marriage was to keep other people "out of the bedroom." This meant it is really no one else's business how and when you and your spouse decide to expand your family. Friends and family mean well, but not everyone will be able to wrap his or her mind around the decision to have someone else carry your child— even if it is genetically your egg and your husband's sperm. You owe no explanations; you can only hope that people will simply be happy for you both. Generally, people will be curious. This is especially true if you are the first within your family, group of friends, or workplace to embark on this journey. Take it in stride, assume positive intent, and make family and friends as comfortable about the process as you have become.

Those who are closest to you will know about your physical and emotional battles with infertility and will be very excited when they hear you are expecting. I hope *Stork's Journey* encourages you as you seek the right way for your family.

CHAPTER 2

The Due Diligence Process

WHEN YOU DECIDE not to go through an agency, you become your own agency. You must take the lead to coordinate things amongst everyone involved in the process. You will manage the activities and information between the surrogate, the attorney(s), the fertility clinic(s), the ob-gyn, and the hospital. This requires effort and good organizational skills to ensure things progress and are on track. In the case of all parties and entities involved, you must choose carefully. After all, you have a lot at stake. Before you can manage activities and information, however, you need to choose the following: the state where your surrogacy process will happen, an attorney, and your gestational surrogate.

Regarding your choice of fertility clinics, ob-gyns, and hospitals, consider leveraging your personal experience and the knowledge you have acquired along the journey. If you are reading my book, chances are you're already familiar with fertility clinics and have had at least one round of IVF. You might have been pregnant at least once. In my case, I moved thousands of miles away from where my embryos were created and stored. I knew I would not be using this clinic for the embryo transfer. I knew I was working with an experienced surrogate, so I spoke with her about the clinics she had used in the past. After some discussion about the best clinic to use for our embryo transfer, I opted to use the clinic she highly recommended. (It also happened to be twenty-five minutes away from her home.) I had my embryos shipped there for the transfer. I was quite pleased with the service and care we received before and after the transfer. In the case of the ob-gyn as well as the hospital, I chose my surrogate's recommendations. I have no regrets about selecting the ob-gyn or the hospital based on my surrogate's recommendations. However, you might have other factors and considerations that sway your decision. If your surrogate lives in another state and you want her to give birth in the state where you reside, then this has to be discussed very early in the process—before attorneys get involved. This will determine whether you retain an attorney in your home state or whether you retain an attorney in her home state. The surrogacy laws vary state to state; therefore, you will need to understand and know what is required (legally) for you to proceed and meet the obligations of the agreement.

Surrogacy Laws and Choosing an Attorney

US surrogacy laws vary from state and state. Starting out, you'll need to find important information about your state's surrogacy laws. Some states are more surrogate friendly than others. In some states, surrogacy is outright forbidden. Anyone who enters into a surrogacy agreement in those states could be fined $10,000 or more. At the time of publication, Arizona, Michigan, New York, and Washington, DC, all have laws or statutes that forbid surrogacy. In the case of other states, there might be stipulations, such as the intended parents needing to be married. The surrogacy agreements might also be unenforceable. Since laws change over time, you will need to know and understand the surrogacy laws based on when and where you decide to start the process. Online resources are available for your education and information. I would suggest searching for the phrase "US surrogacy laws."

For more information, you can also consult an attorney who practices surrogacy law. Your surrogate, if she is experienced, might be able to provide a referral for an attorney—especially if she has worked with one for past arrangements. However, your surrogate might not have a complete understanding of the legal activities affiliated with the surrogacy process. Her interaction with the attorney might have been limited (if her interaction was through an agency). Therefore, before retaining an attorney, make sure you take time to see whether the attorney has any reviews online from past clients or from the surrogacy community. The attorney's service and responsiveness could vary depending on whether he or she is working with an agency (where he or she stands to lose hundreds of current and future clients) or whether he or she is just working with you. Some attorneys have reputations for being extremely slow—bordering on unprofessionalism. Moreover, if the attorney is not on top of things, there could be personal and legal implications as well as costly delays.

Understanding US surrogacy laws from state to state will guide your decision in selecting an attorney and a gestational surrogate. It is important to note that your choice of attorney will depend on where your potential surrogate lives. Remember, the attorney must be licensed to practice law in the state where the surrogate resides and/or will give birth to your child. The attorney will be responsible for drafting the gestational surrogacy agreement that you will have in place with your surrogate. In addition, the attorney will ensure the agreement is filed with the applicable courts and that a prebirth order is secured in a timely manner. This will help avoid any confusion at the hospital after the birth of your child.

Choosing a Surrogate

Whether you turn to a family member, friend, or stranger as a surrogate, you will need to decide how deep a relationship you will have with your surrogate. Keep in mind, though, it must be comprehensive enough to determine whether you and the surrogate are a good match and that things will go as smoothly as possible during the entire process.

It's important that you are in tune with your emotional intelligence when selecting a surrogate. If you sense or see a few things that do not quite sit well with you early in the screening process, do not sweep them under the rug. Address them openly. This way, you make the best possible decision in selecting a surrogate.

Typically, this is a business arrangement in which you have negotiated a monetary sum and other related terms with your surrogate. However, human nature is involved, and the surrogacy process can become overly complex if key expectations are not reviewed and agreed upon up front. For intended parents, surrogacy might be the last option and chance to have children who are genetically related. Thus, some (or even most) intended parents might strongly prefer to have only surface and transactional relationships with surrogates. This sentiment might be a result of the parents feeling a bit resentful that they could not carry their own child. They also might want to preserve their emotions for the baby and not share as much emotional energy with the surrogate. Some intended parents might not want any further contact with the surrogate after birth. Other intended parents might not know what kind of relationship they want postbirth and would rather let their journey with the surrogate guide them. This is all fine. However, you need to have these important conversations with your surrogate before embryo transfer. These conversations should occur while you are still trying to decide whether this person is the right surrogate match for you.

Since you have decided (or will be deciding) on whether or not to work through a surrogacy agency, you must know there are alternate means of finding a suitable surrogate. One great website I mentioned in the previous chapter is Surromomsonline.com. As with anything online, you need to do your due diligence in vetting the process and the potential surrogate. Take your time; this is such an important, costly, and life-altering experience. You should spend several weeks to several months screening potential surrogates. Do so until you feel comfortable enough to move on to the next steps in the selection process. Do not ever let a surrogate rush you to commit because of her personal situation. For example, she might be at a crossroads with her insurance because of an employment change for someone in her household. She might have had another set of intended parents fall through, or she might simply be desperate for income. Don't give in! This is your journey and your baby. You will want to ensure you do everything possible to make the process anxiety and stress-free.

If you decide against using an agency, you will need a greater degree of trust and respect between you, your partner, and the gestational surrogate. For example, when I narrowed it down to two surrogates, one was within my state, and another was outside my state. The final decision came down to trust. The surrogate within my state had worked with surrogacy agencies in the past and had decided to go independent around the time she answered my ad. In doing so, she had not realized she would need to be more forthcoming with me about her personal information. When I asked for her social security number to perform a background check, she declined. She wanted to give the information to the attorney (whom I would have used had I selected a surrogate in my own state). She tried to contact my attorney at the time, but my attorney never returned her e-mails or calls. My lawyer reminded me that I had retained her for legal services and she would have no dealings with the surrogate. Moreover, my attorney advised that if the surrogate was noncompliant, I should move on to someone else. I did give the potential surrogate the opportunity to perform her own background check, but she declined. At that point, I decided to go with the surrogate who resided in a different but still surrogate-friendly state.

Screening Surrogates

As you begin to screen potential surrogates, it is important to ask questions that are fundamental to the process. Even if the surrogate answers the questions favorably for your situation, you should make an extra effort to get to know each potential surrogate's personality and disposition. There is so much a psychological evaluation report is not able to tell you about a surrogate's personality—how she thinks, views the world, and deals with stressful situations. To try to get some of these answers, you can ask the surrogate to take a personality test (e.g., the Jung Typology Test or the Myers-Briggs Type Indicator) in addition to a psychological examination. You will need to be familiar with personality and style assessments to understand the results and what they might mean for you during the entire surrogacy process. There are no good or bad personality types. Having information about the

Personality Type test will put you in the best position to understand how to communicate and relate with your Surrogate throughout the pregnancy. Basically, you need to get to know one another as much as you can before you decide to transfer your very precious embryo(s) into this person.

Questions to Ask

Whether a potential surrogate is someone who answers your ad or someone you know (a family member, friend, or acquaintance), when you are considering entrusting her with carrying your child, you can never ask too many questions. The kinds of things that come up when she is already carrying your child will surprise you and will likely be things you wish you had known ahead of time. I've included a list of helpful questions to ask a potential surrogate about her thoughts on the surrogacy process, health, and wellness. The questions also cover her family and homelife. Besides the questions listed below, feel free to add your own questions based on your personal situation.

Surrogacy Process

1. How old are you?
2. When would you be ready to start?
3. What was the date of your last delivery? (Ideally, a surrogate should wait at least six to seven months after delivery to allow the uterus and body to heal.)
4. Do you have an IVF clinic in _____ (state) that you have used for past IVF treatments and embryo transfers?
5. What is your requested base compensation, and what does it include?
6. Are you open to carrying multiples (e.g., twins or triplets) for us?
7. Have your deliveries been natural or C-section?
8. How many pregnancies have you had?
9. Have you had any miscarriages with any pregnancies?

10. How long have you been an independent gestational surrogate?
11. What have your experiences been like with prior intended parents?
12. Do you have medical insurance? If so, how much does it cover? Does it cover IVF, IVF medications, or embryo transfers?
    - Would you be able to provide a copy of your medical insurance plan/coverage? We need to understand whether there are any exclusions.
13. Do you carry supplemental insurance? If so, with whom? What is the coverage?
14. Will you honor our privacy and confidentiality, which are important to us? Contractually, we ask you not to post any pictures of yourself while carrying our child or discuss our surrogacy arrangement on social media or anywhere on the Internet. Do you agree?
15. Is there a fertility clinic or hospital you have used in the past through the surrogacy process that you would recommend?
16. Do you have a recent letter (from the past six months) from your ob-gyn or fertility clinic clearing you to become a surrogate?
17. Have you had a mental or psychological screening completed to indicate you are mentally fit to undertake this process?
18. What are your beliefs on selective reduction or termination?
19. Are you willing to go through a background check? Do you already have on file a background check from a certified and reputable agency from within the last six months that you can provide?
20. Are you familiar with the surrogacy laws in your state?
21. What are your biggest fears or concerns regarding the surrogacy process?
22. What is your preference on communication and involvement from the intended parents during the pregnancy?
23. How do you feel about contact and/or a relationship with us and our child post birth?
24. Would you be willing to pump breast milk for _____ (period of time)? Please explain or elaborate.

Health, Wellness, and Safety

25. How would you describe your overall health, diet/nutrition, and lifestyle?
26. What is your body mass index (BMI)?
27. Are you a smoker or drinker?
28. Do you use or have you ever used recreational drugs?
29. Have you ever been diagnosed with depression or bipolar disorder?
30. Do you consider yourself an emotional person?
31. Are you on any prescribed medications? Do you take any herbal or vitamin supplements? If so, what?
32. Do you get sick or ill frequently (e.g., cold, coughs, fatigue, etc.)?
33. Have you ever been diagnosed with a serious illness in your lifetime?
34. Have you had any major surgeries or procedures over the past ten years?
35. Do you have a family history of blood disorders, diabetes, or high blood pressure?
36. Were you or have you ever been on bed rest or pelvic rest for any recent pregnancies? If so, please explain.
37. Have you ever discontinued your employment (on doctor's orders) because of issues with pregnancy?
38. Do you agree to never consume artificial sweeteners during our pregnancy and avoid personal-care products with parabens?
39. Do you have any tattoos or body piercings? How many? Where?
40. Do you have an active life-insurance policy?
41. Do you or does anyone in your household own and/or carry any firearms? Please explain.

Family and Homelife

42. How would you describe your homelife/environment?
43. What are your personal values and beliefs?
44. Are you employed? Do you work full or part time? What's the nature of your profession?

45. If you are not employed, is surrogacy the only form of income for your household?
46. Are you married, partnered, or single?
47. If you are married or living with a partner, do you feel safe in your marriage and in your home?
48. If you are married or partnered, does your spouse/partner work outside of the home?
49. How does your family feel about the surrogacy process?
50. Do you have a support system in place (friends or family) that you can rely on as you go through the surrogacy process?
51. What are your hobbies and interests?
52. How do you handle stress and stressful situations?
53. Are you a foster parent? Does anyone else live in your home besides your birth child (or children) and spouse? If so, why?
54. What is your highest level of education?
55. What is your spouse's highest level of education?
56. Will you be honest, reliable, and dependable? You must be someone who takes initiative when necessary but who will also consult us when needed. Do you agree?
57. What is your personality type? Please take the Jung Typology Test (also known as the Myers-Briggs Type Indicator, or MBTI). The test can be found here: http://www.humanmetrics.com/cgi-win/jtypes2.asp.

I chose an experienced surrogate. When she carried my child, it was her third time being a gestational surrogate. While I had a learning curve, it was not as steep as it would have been if I had worked with a first-time gestational surrogate. My surrogate educated me on various aspects of the process, which helped a lot.

Contracts

You will want to ensure you have the following documents in hand before you have an attorney draft a gestational surrogacy agreement. In some cases, you might have to pay for these documents since you have the vested interest.

1. A background check on your surrogate.
2. A home study of your surrogate. You will want to understand her home environment in terms of whether it is safe and secure during pregnancy.
3. A valid medical clearance letter from your surrogate's primary physician.
4. A valid surrogacy clearance letter for your surrogate from a reputable fertility clinic.
5. A psychological examination from a licensed psychologist.
6. A copy of your surrogate's current insurance policy, which should provide medical coverage throughout the pregnancy. You will need to understand the exclusions in the policy. You need to understand whether you will need to carry supplemental insurance.

You should discuss all your must-haves with your potential surrogate before signing any agreements. In some cases, you might want to have contractual protection by building certain requirements into the contract.

For example, you might have a strict diet and want your surrogate to follow the same diet or avoid certain types of beverages or foods. You will need to agree with the surrogate on this up front. If she is willing—but it would be vastly different from her current diet or the change would be a bit of an inconvenience—you might have to work out some type of arrangement with her. You could decide to order food and mail it to her or make some other type of financial concession.

You might also have strict policies on personal grooming, such as avoiding hair dyeing, gel pedicures or manicures, or personal-care products with certain chemicals (e.g., parabens).

Here's the truth though. Unless you have a live-in surrogate, it will be difficult to monitor your surrogate every day to ensure she's following your required guidelines and requests. There must be a great deal of trust between you and your surrogate. No one is perfect, and each day brings its own set of challenges. Depending on how your surrogate is feeling and what other things she might be experiencing, there might be days where she forgets or lets your requirements lapse. What's important is to ensure you have the kind of relationship where she is comfortable enough to confide in you about her shortcomings, frustrations, and concerns regarding the pregnancy and your expectations. With a strong relationship of mutual respect, you'll be able to work together on the best course of action.

This stage may seem overwhelming or daunting. It is very manageable. Be thoughtful in your approach because laying this groundwork should allow for a more positive surrogacy process.

CHAPTER 3

Get Organized!

ONCE YOU HAVE selected your surrogate, it's time to get organized. You will need to determine how frequently you should be corresponding with your attorney. You will need to understand what the major legal milestones are throughout the process. Be diligent about planning the doctor appointments and a focused meeting/visit at the hospital prebirth.

Financial Matters

You might decide to set up an escrow account to remit payment to your surrogate. Typically, the escrow account will cost you a few hundred or a few thousand dollars above and beyond the payment schedule outlined with the surrogate. This might be a requirement, but it depends on the surrogate or the attorney. Otherwise, you can either use an existing bank account or set up a new bank account specifically for this arrangement. You will need to ensure you pay your surrogate on time. These payments will be based on the schedule your attorney outlined in the gestational surrogacy agreement. In most cases, payment is every four weeks.

I was very fortunate that my surrogate worked full time and genuinely cared about helping another family. She was not out to nickel-and-dime me at every turn. When I was screening surrogates, some potential candidates seemed to want a fee at every turn, which felt exploitive of our plight. I get it. It's a business arrangement, and intended parents are at the mercy of supply and demand. Still, the delicacy of the situation should warrant some consideration on the part of the surrogate.

Please note that besides the negotiated compensation with your surrogate, you will probably be responsible for her out-of-pocket medical expenses relating to the pregnancy. You will need to set aside funds for that as well. Below is an example of the major expenses related to the whole surrogacy process:

1. Base compensation—paid to the surrogate
2. Upcharge fee for multiples—paid to the surrogate
3. Maternity clothes allowance—paid to the surrogate
4. Attorney costs and legal fees—paid to the attorney
5. Psychological evaluation costs (for both the surrogate and intended parents)
6. Out-of-pocket medical costs (after insurance) during pregnancy and delivery
7. Travel costs for the surrogate and intended parents
8. Embryo transfer and medication costs

Depending on your situation, it is important to know that other costs might be incurred. Besides the out-of-pocket medical costs, the standard GC agreement might accommodate the surrogate in specific circumstances. For example, there might be a payout of several hundred dollars to a few thousand dollars for selective termination, dilation and curettage, amniocentesis, cervical cerclage, or loss of reproductive organs. You might be required to secure a life insurance policy for your surrogate in anticipation of pregnancy. Should your surrogate be medically mandated to go on bed rest, you might be subject to a bed-rest fee, and you might be liable for lost salary and wages should your surrogate's employment status be impacted. It is critical you read your surrogacy agreement carefully and that your attorney best represents your interests. In most cases, there is also a cost for having your surrogate provide breast milk for your newborn. The rate is negotiable, but typically it ranges from a few cents to a few dollars per ounce. Additionally, there could be travel expenses for both you and the surrogate. If the surrogate has children, she might want you to cover childcare costs for when she's away at appointments relating to the pregnancy. Discussions with your attorney and the surrogate can help you determine the fees and costs you will need to cover.

Surrogacy can be quite costly. There are financing options which cover reproduction health expenses (IVF, surrogacy) that are available through clinics and other 3rd party companies. Simple searches online can yield in great resources for you to explore. Again, I was blessed to have been able to afford it without financing or going into debt. The cost for gestational surrogacy (including all agency fees, attorneys' fees, screening and surrogate fees, and medical and insurance costs) can range from around $100,000 to $150,000, depending on varying services and fees that may be required for each individual situation.

All costs considered, my expenses were nearly half of the cost figure at the lower end of the range. I tracked everything meticulously on spreadsheets....every expense incurred! Nearly half of the total costs is the compensation that you will pay the surrogate. Negotiating the base compensation with the potential surrogate is critical. Taking the lead and being in a position to negotiate does not necessarily mean that you are compromising the quality of the surrogate or the quality of the experience. This is where spending time upfront vetting surrogates and getting to know their motivations are fundamental. Moreover, forgoing the Surrogacy Agency route eliminates a lot of the "overhead" costs associated with this process. You can definitely do this!

In the Doctor's Office: Paperwork and Appointments

Before your surrogate goes to any doctor's appointments, you will need to make sure your name is on your surrogate's HIPAA forms (as it relates to the pregnancy). Have your surrogate confirm you are listed on her HIPAA forms at the fertility clinic before the embryo transfer. Confirm also with her ob-gyn's office. This will ensure you can contact the medical providers directly if you have questions or if you are concerned about the pregnancy for any reason.

Depending on your personal situation, you might want to attend all appointments or a few selected appointments. Make plans either way. To keep my costs low, I chose to visit my out-of-state surrogate for milestone appointments. This included the eight-week ultrasound and an appointment with maternal-fetal medicine (high-risk pregnancy experts) at thirty-one weeks, during which I worked in a meeting with the hospital to make sure things were in place before delivery. I made plans to travel to my surrogate for the twenty-week anatomy scan, but due to inclement weather, my flight was canceled. For all other appointments with the ob-gyn (one every four weeks), I joined via Skype. It was no more than twenty minutes during the workday every four weeks, so I marked it on my calendar.

Even though your surrogate is carrying the baby, the responsibility of knowing what is going on with the pregnancy should not reside solely with her. From the time your surrogate begins the embryo transfer process, you should know and understand her medical protocol (medications, doses, and frequency). If a positive pregnancy results, you should keep track of the surrogate's HCG (a hormone produced after implantation) levels to ensure the pregnancy is progressing well for the first several weeks after it is confirmed. Make a note of the fetus's heartbeat at every appointment, and make sure you track the weight and body measurements provided to you during the ultrasounds. Always come prepared with questions to ask the medical providers.

Also, you need to confirm that you, the medical providers (obstetrician and maternal-fetal specialist), and your surrogate are on the same page regarding any medication and vaccination protocols throughout the pregnancy. Since the nurses at the ob-gyn office usually administer the medications and vaccines after the ultrasound appointments, make sure you ask the doctor about medications and vaccines during the appointment. If you are not able to make the appointment in person or via video conference, bring it up in conversation with your surrogate. You might want to make it clear with your surrogate that the decision to take medication or receive vaccines should be discussed with you before any medication is administered.

I was able to attend the thirty-one-week appointment in person. I did this for different reasons. First, I had not seen my surrogate since the eight-week appointment, and with the preterm labor scare during the twenty-seventh week, I wanted the satisfaction of being there in person and knowing things were progressing as they should. Since my daughter was going to be born via surrogate, I decided to schedule a visit with the hospital to ensure everything on the day of her birth and during my daughter's hospital stay would proceed without a hitch. During the hospital visit, I met with the patient relations coordinator, the head of the maternity ward, and the coordinator of patient records for one hour or so. We discussed the activities leading up to and after the birth of my daughter. Even though my surrogate was giving birth, we were still our daughter's parents. Given the safety and security measures of any maternity ward, we wanted to ensure we complied with hospital policies, but we also wanted to ensure we were given the proper consideration.

On the day of my daughter's birth, we were given wristbands with the name of my surrogate. This gave us the privilege to come in and out of the maternity ward. We were given a separate hospital room where we could start bonding with our daughter when she wasn't in the nursery undergoing the first medical screens for newborns. Since my surrogate was scheduled for a C-section, my husband and I were able to plan our travel and ensure we would be there for our daughter's birth and up to one week afterward. There were no confusions at the hospital as to why we were there, and we were catered to as the rightful parents.

Your Involvement and the Surrogate

All intended parents are different in terms of how engaged they will be in the process. It depends on their financial resources, their work and home situations, and distance from the surrogates. Never let the surrogate make you feel guilty if you do not keep the same schedule as the intended parents before you. For me, it was more important to make sure my surrogate received the full compensation as outlined in our surrogacy agreement. I had to budget and plan accordingly. While I'm sure my surrogate would have wanted me to attend every appointment, I did not see this as essential to the process.

Decide how and in what manner you will communicate with your surrogate. For example, how often will you check in by text message rather than having a phone conversation? This could evolve over time, but decide on a minimum with the surrogate. You can build from there. For me, I texted my surrogate every morning, but we spoke by phone at least once per week. Outside of this established frequency, we were both welcome to pick up the phone and reach one another if it was necessary or important. Some intended parents might want to talk to the surrogate every day or perhaps twice daily. Do what works best for both parties.

Although there are many plans to make, you will be able to accomplish all you need to with intentional, respectful communication with the attorneys, doctors, and surrogate.

CHAPTER 4

Creating Healthy Boundaries

CREATING AND MAINTAINING healthy boundaries with your surrogate throughout the surrogacy process is important. Again, boundaries and the surrogate/parent relationship should be discussed up front—before any surrogacy agreements are signed and before any embryo is transferred.

For some intended parents, surrogacy is the last and only option. It is, therefore, understandable that some might prefer to have a transactional type of relationship. They might want to move on with their lives with no further relationship with the surrogate postbirth.

For most, becoming a surrogate is a very rewarding and fulfilling experience. The surrogate might have a natural inclination to want the intended parents to be fully involved and engaged throughout the process. This is a great opportunity for the intended parents to influence the process and possibly make a lifelong friend.

Contractual Relationship to Friendship

Somewhere and somehow, the intended parents and the surrogate must come to an understanding. Contractually (based on the surrogacy agreement), there is no obligation for the intended parents to become friends with the surrogate or to have contact with her postbirth. This desire has to develop naturally between the two parties. While there should be a very respectful and cordial relationship with your surrogate, you should exercise discernment and discretion in what information you disclose to her about your life. At the end of the day, surrogacy does not mean you relinquish the right to keep your life and marriage private. On the other hand, you are paying the surrogate, and she is carrying your child. Therefore, there must be less privacy on her side in terms of the arrangement. You have the right to ask about her lifestyle and activities to the extent that it might impact your child in any manner. You might become close friends with your surrogate, but let this happen naturally. If it is forced for either party, the outcome could be disappointing, and you'll sense the tension and strain in the relationship.

Communication and Privacy

Discuss communication if you sense your surrogate is prone to wanting or needing attention. For example, if your surrogate's lifestyle affords her the time to text frequently, but your lifestyle (due to work or personal preference) does not, discuss communication frequency up front. Initially, my surrogate was texting me throughout the day. I did not want her to feel as though I was being dismissive or that I did not want to communicate with her. I was heavily involved in business meetings or on conference calls and would not be able to engage in frequent text correspondences with her throughout the day. I informed her I would text her daily though—usually in the morning before I left for work and sometimes in the evenings after I got home. Unless we had an appointment that day (which I would be joining via Skype) or had to correspond about pertinent surrogacy business, I would not be responding to text messages during the workday.

You will also need to discuss privacy and confidentiality if those things are important to you. For example, some intended parents decide not to inform their children they were born via surrogacy and do not want any evidence (online or otherwise) that could violate that wish. You might want to ask your surrogate not to mention your names or post any pictures or stories about the process. You can work with your attorney to factor this into your contract if this is critical for you. Please note that if your surrogate gives birth in a different state from where you live, the child's birth certificate will list the state and city where the child was delivered. Hence, even if you attempt to shield your child from the surrogacy process, questions could arise in the future regarding his or her place of birth relative to where you were residing at that time.

The surrogate might ask you questions that seem intrusive and too familiar for the kind of relationship you want with this individual. She likely means no harm. She might be curious, and she could be trying to develop a stronger relationship or bond with you by getting to know you more personally. There are several ways to address this. Keep the lines of communication open. You can decide to have a heart-to-heart with your surrogate about boundaries. Again, this should be discussed before you sign the surrogacy agreement. However, if you are a first-time intended parent, it might take time for you to determine how much of your life you are willing to share with your surrogate.

Emotional Support

While the psychological evaluation is proof the surrogate is mentally fit to undertake the surrogacy process, what some intended parents do not consider or prepare for is an experienced gestational surrogate who might need reassurance and emotional support from you along the way.

Keep in mind that the surrogate is carrying your baby. She will want to know you care about the process and about the fact she is undertaking the care of your child. While you might feel this is a given, a little reassurance might be comforting to her. This might mean following up with her a little more diligently (but empathetically) if she's not feeling well or if there are some general concerns regarding the pregnancy.

To make the process joyous and comfortable for your surrogate, consider things you can do or buy for her (and for your baby). For example, I purchased a full-body pillow for my surrogate so she could have more restful sleep as her belly grew. I purchased a neck pillow and some decaffeinated fruit teas for her. I made sure I remembered her birthday and took her out to lunch on my visits. I provided plenty of prenatal vitamins for her (the ones I preferred), and I made my payments to her in a timely manner. I kept all the promises I had made from the beginning to gain and build her trust. Again, I was in touch with her daily.

After the Baby Is Born

Before your child is born, you will need to decide and discuss whether you want the surrogate to hold the baby after birth or while the baby is still in the hospital. This can be a very sensitive issue with all parties involved. The intended parents will likely want the opportunity to develop a strong bond with their child immediately after the birth. You will need to discuss boundaries with the surrogate ahead of time in order to avoid awkward situations for both parties at the hospital. What will you allow the surrogate to do or not do postbirth? Will you allow her to visit you and the child during the baby's hospital stay? You might feel you want some alone time with your partner and the baby (as a family unit) without interference from the surrogate. The surrogate, however, might want to visit the baby, needing some type of closure from the process. Among other things, you will have to decide if you will allow her to breastfeed your child or if she will pump breast milk for the first few days. Give serious thought to what you want postbirth. If you feel different after the child is born, it's OK. This is such a life-altering event that you cannot predict your emotions ahead of time.

The first couple weeks postbirth are exciting but also challenging. Your newborn will be feeding every two to three hours within a twenty-four-hour period. This means your normal sleep pattern will be altered, and you will have to adjust accordingly. Getting to know your newborn, understanding his or her needs, and forging a parent-child bond are critical during the first few weeks. You might want your space and privacy to do this without contact from the surrogate, your family, or your friends. There might be a psychological and emotional desire to disconnect from your surrogate as you start your new life with your baby. However, you might also welcome contact with the surrogate if you need a sense of closure. You might find you welcome visits and help from family and friends. It's entirely up to you.

Healthy boundaries make healthy relationships. It is vital to maintain those boundaries that will keep you feeling emotionally secure—especially at this special time and in this unconventional relationship with your surrogate. It's important to let the bond and the relationship develop and strengthen naturally.

Plan, Plan, and Plan

PROPER PLANNING IS paramount! In addition to your due diligence at the beginning of the process, it is important for you to conduct your due diligence in terms of how the surrogacy process will or could impact your life. As you excitedly wait for the baby to arrive, it's time to plan to take time off work and prepare your home (and yourself) for your newest family member's arrival.

Taking Time Off, Maternity Leave, or a Leave of Absence

As soon as you can, you should investigate your employer's policy regarding maternity leave for a surrogacy arrangement. In most cases, since you are not physically giving birth, there is no medical reason for you to be on short-term disability according to company leave policy. Therefore, in the instances of adoption or surrogacy, short-term disability is usually not an option. You might be surprised to learn you may have to use your allocated vacation days at the start of your leave period. After that, you will need to go on leave, as per the Family and Medical Leave Act (FMLA). While you might have expected some percentage of your salary to be paid through several weeks if you went on short-term disability, FMLA leave is completely unpaid. In addition to all the money you spend on surrogacy, you will need to make a plan to account for the adjusted income during your maternity leave period. It is better to find out about the maternity leave policy early in the surrogacy process. This insight will help you budget for time off, appropriately. As you will want medical coverage while you are on leave, if applicable, you will need to investigate medical coverage options and payments under COBRA. Additionally, you should contact your insurance company and understand the process by which medical coverage would be extended to your child after birth (premature or full term). If your child should require substantial and extensive medical care post birth, especially if he or she is preterm, you should understand the exclusion in your medical coverage.

Your employer might offer adoption assistance or something similar. This can be as little as $5,000. You should find out if that assistance also applies to surrogacy. In my case, it did not.

You should inform your manager, team, and HR representative about your pregnancy so that they are aware of this life-altering event. You will want their support and cooperation if you need to travel for appointments and other work-related reasons. Should your baby be born preterm (before thirty-seven weeks), you would not want to surprise your manager by informing him or her about this pregnancy for the first time at that point. Also, you will want to make sure you and your manager have agreed on your coverage plan for when you are on maternity leave.

Also, if you and your spouse or partner must return to work after two to three months, it would be a good idea to start looking into childcare options well before your baby is born. If you don't have a family member or friend who can watch your child during the workday, start exploring the costs and advantages and disadvantages of day care, au pairs, babysitting, and nanny services.

Surrogacy can be quite costly. Even with the high cost and complexity of this untraditional method of expanding a family, payments to the surrogate are not tax deductible. However, medical expenses incurred by the sperm and egg donor are tax deductible (including IVF expenses, doctor visits, lab fees, and medication). For tax guidance, please consult a tax accountant, tax attorney, or other tax professional.

Getting Yourself Ready

To stay abreast of everything going on during this exciting time in your life, you might want to begin journaling about the process –which can be cathartic for you. In addition, you will want to register with BabyCenter.

com or TheBump.com. Otherwise, you can download the apps for those sites. In either case, these resources will help you stay in tune with the fetus's week-to-week developmental milestones. In addition, there are great resources available about what you will need to know or purchase as the pregnancy progresses. After the first trimester, I made purchases with every monthly milestone. I was in full blown nesting mode.

While you aren't physically carrying the baby, there is nothing that prevents you from reading as much as you can about caring for your newborn child. Spend the last several weeks of the pregnancy reading. For further preparation, sign up for childcare or newborn classes at your local hospital four to six weeks before the birth of your child. Consider signing up for CPR and safety classes as well.

Preparing the Home & Lifestyle

You might receive baby furniture from your family, or you might decide to purchase some baby furniture at a garage sale. However, if you decide to purchase new, you could be looking at a four- to twelve-week lead time. The same could be true for a custom glider (nursery rocking chair), a dresser, or any other major nursery furniture. Plan accordingly. Some things you will need for the baby have longer lead times than others. Make sure you make timely decisions on purchases so you have everything you need before the baby arrives.

If you live in a cold weather/snowy climate, ideally you would want to have an all-wheel-drive or four-wheel-drive vehicle. It would be terrible to get stuck in the snow with your newborn baby in the car. It is never a pleasant experience trying to dig out of the snow, pushing the car, and having others help. Can you imagine doing all that with a baby in the car who is exposed to the risk of cold and other danger? Similarly, if you live in a warmer area, consider getting the appropriate car-window tints that would protect the baby from UVA and UVB rays and heat exposure, and make sure your car's air-conditioning system is fully functional.

When people hear you are expecting, one thing they will often say is, "Be prepared to never sleep again." This comment is a bit odd, but it should motivate you to get ready for the baby since your discretionary time will be scarce. This means decluttering closets and storage, cleaning throughout the house, painting, and completing house projects. Consider stocking up on bottled water, paper goods, and personal items (toilet paper, paper towels, paper plates, plastic cups, soap, toothpaste, razors, shampoo, conditioner, laundry detergent, etc.). In previous eras, stores did not offer mail or in-person delivery. With the creation of these services, the lives of new parents can be a lot less stressful. If you can find a few minutes to order the things you need online, the services and goods come to you. With a baby on the way, I hired a housekeeper to help with the deep cleaning and decluttering. I purchased an adequate supply of disposable plates and cups to minimize the time and worry of dishwashing the first three months. It was worth it for us. Although there are a lot of things to think about, the more planning you do (and the more you accomplish of what you plan), the more smoothly everything will go when the baby comes home.

CHAPTER 6

The Whiteboard—YOLO

THAT'S RIGHT. YOLO—YOU only live once!

Surrogacy is a blessing! As intended parents, it is easy to get immersed in the process, and you should. However, don't miss out on the opportunity to take a step back, take a deep breath, and realize you should seize the experience of being physically unencumbered.

Take advantage of more frequent quality time with your spouse. Once the baby arrives, your marriage will change. If there is a trip or vacation you have been planning for years, this might be the time to take this trip. I know—surrogacy already costs a lot of money, so you might not be able to afford a luxury vacation. Think about a few weekend getaways with your spouse, family, or friends. Consider trying a hobby or interest you have always wanted to try. Go to the movies, enjoy your favorite restaurants, try new restaurants, get in shape (or in better shape), learn a language, or fulfill some deferred dream. Is there a surgical or medical procedure you've been delaying? Are you due for a doctor or dentist appointment? This is the time to get these personal projects completed. Once the baby arrives, you will need plenty of stamina and energy. You will want to be at optimal health.

Just because you are expecting a baby doesn't mean life is over. However, life will change once the baby is born, and your discretionary time will be significantly limited for quite some time. Live it up now!

Having this time before the baby arrives is like having a virtual whiteboard. It's like having a clean space to realize dreams or deferred goals. Anything you can think of relative to this whiteboard—any hope, dream, or trip you've been putting off—you now have express permission to do.

What would you want to do or see? Since it is your life, you need not feel guilty about it or disclose any of it to your surrogate.

Giving careful thought about time spent before the baby arrives is critical in helping you and your partner feel better prepared as a couple and as individuals. These fun and fulfilling activities could help strengthen you and your marriage. They also help build anticipation for the arrival of the little one.

CHAPTER 7

The Road Less Traveled

MY LITTLE GIRL was born on a warm summer morning in an area nestled among the most rugged brown mountains of Provo, Utah. I could not fall asleep the night before her birth because of the sheer excitement and nervousness that I felt. As ready as I felt for her arrival, I could not have imagined the utter joy, happiness, and relief I felt when I heard her cry for the first time. She was born healthy and into a figurative covering of prayers and well-wishes that I had taken time to write weeks in advance. It was important for me to utter blessings on my child just a few minutes after her arrival into our world. Those few days in the hospital were surreal. I had waited such a long time to become a mother, so I was overjoyed and delighted to hold her and tend to her every need.

Everything for which I had labored and prayed came to fruition. The planning, the organization, and the due diligence had all paid off. There were days after I brought her home that I thought I should have gone through the experience sooner, but in reality, it happened for us at the right time.

With so many women and couples struggling with infertility, more and more people may take the road less traveled. In time, the road less traveled might become a main road of some sort. Even being blessed with the option of gestational surrogacy, my sincere wish is that more time and money would be poured into really understanding the true cause and cure of uterine fibroids…and other related causes of Infertility. For us, this road of surrogacy has made all the difference in our lives. We are so in love with our daughter. She is the most beautiful and happy baby. We are humbled at the thought of welcoming her sister or brother at the right time in the future by this same process.

Stay encouraged! You can do this.

Here's hoping that the stork lands on your doorstep. All the best on your journey!

CHAPTER 8

Husband's Excerpt

IF SURROGACY WAS the only choice we had, I thought to myself, *Why not try?* Was I comfortable with it at the beginning? Absolutely not! After researching and reading about other people who had gone through the process though, I realized we were not alone. After all, it was still our embryo. *Why not?* I thought again. What did we have to lose?

My wife did a great job as she took on the role of the agency and the real role as the intended parent! If it hadn't been for her diligence and determined spirit, I would not have gone through with surrogacy. I was very worried about what would happen following the birth of our daughter (rather than the months leading up to her birth). I really didn't want our daughter to find out how she was born. I was concerned our child would find out about the process and not understand all her mother and I had gone through to bring her into this world. In some ways, I was afraid of all the questions she would have in addition to any judgments she would make. Would she be satisfied with knowing we were her true biological parents, or would she develop a desire to find her surrogate carrier—as if she felt a missing link in her life? Honestly, I did not want to keep in touch with the surrogate and her husband. Even though the surrogate's decision to carry our child was seemingly heroic and gracious on their part, I felt they were adequately compensated. It was not as if they were doing it for free. I felt that compensation was fulfilled and contractual obligations were met.

Getting Organized

In terms of getting organized for the process, I tried to accept that surrogacy was the way we had to do things. I was more than ready to have a child, and surrogacy did not make me feel any different in that respect. My uncertainties and questions revolved around the relationship with the surrogate postbirth. I knew that life would be completely different once the baby arrived, and I sensed that life would change for the better. Some individuals often make it seem as if life is over or will be really hard once a child arrives. I try to see life and things in a much more upbeat and positive manner. I believed the baby would make our marriage stronger. I was focused on making preparations to create financial stability to provide the baby everything he or she would need.

Creating Healthy Boundaries

I was certain I wanted to meet the surrogate. After all, we would be entrusting this woman with the most precious job in the world…the job of carrying our child. However, I did not want to develop a long-term relationship with the surrogate or her husband. I did have the opportunity to speak to the surrogate on several occasions throughout the thirty-nine weeks. This reassured her I was on board and supportive. I do not feel as if I missed out on the surrogacy experience by not attending the doctor's appointments in person. I was certain I would be present on the day of the child's birth. This was the single most important day for me with regard to the process.

Would I do it again? Well, it depends how things are several months postbirth in terms of our daughter's health and development. Also, we need to wait to see if there will be any adverse situations that surface with the attorney or the surrogate regarding the arrangement. I felt the surrogacy experience might not be concluded after the baby arrived and that there would still be some lingering open doors. However, my wife is one to cross the t's and dot the i's, so I'm certain she made sure everything was settled and concluded. I think I will have a more complete feeling months from now. In due time, the surrogacy process will be a distant memory, and I will only know the joy that my daughter brings me every day.

Despite my reservations about a number of things, including the future possibility of my daughter learning about how she came into this world, I was never embarrassed or ashamed we chose this road. Some of us have to take this path, and you have the distinct privilege of doing the same.

Key Definitions

Gestational Carrier/Gestational Surrogate/Surrogate: These terms are used interchangeably. However, a general surrogate definition is a woman carrying a child for intended parents who are unable to build a family on their own. There are two types of surrogates: traditional surrogates and gestational surrogates.

Intended Parent: Person who becomes the legal parent of a child born through surrogacy.

Gestational Surrogacy: Pregnancy where the surrogate is genetically unrelated to the baby. The embryos are created using the eggs from the intended mother or an egg donor and sperm from the intended father or a sperm donor.

Traditional Surrogacy: Pregnancy where the surrogate is genetically related to the baby and becomes pregnant through artificial insemination. While this used to be common, most surrogacy arrangements today involve gestational surrogacy.

In Vitro Fertilization (IVF): A process by which sperm fertilizes eggs outside the womb in a controlled environment. This is either a test tube or petri dish. A reproductive endocrinologist at an IVF clinic performs the process.

Indie/Indie Surrogate/Indie GC: A surrogate who is not affiliated with a surrogacy agency and works independently to seek intended parents for the purpose of entering into a surrogacy arrangement and agreement.

Frozen Embryo Transfer: A process that occurs when a frozen embryo (an already fertilized and frozen egg) is thawed and transferred into a surrogate.

Carrier Agreement/Surrogacy Contract: A legal contract between the surrogate and intended parents. The parties negotiate the terms of the contract through their legal representation. Once the contract is signed, the terms of the contract govern the parties' interactions. It is very important for the intended parents and the surrogate to read the contract carefully. This way, all terms and conditions are understood.

Egg Retrieval: The process by which eggs are removed from the egg donor for fertilization.

Prebirth Order: A court-issued order acquired before the birth of the child. Typically, it will place the names of the intended parents on the birth certificate and allow the intended parents access to the child while he or she is in the hospital.

Postbirth Order: A court-issued order acquired after the birth of the child. Typically, it will replace the surrogate with the intended parents on the newborn's birth certificate.

Resources/References

The following is a list of resources/references at the time of publication.

Surrogate Mothers Online LLC (http://www.surromomsonline.com)
The goal of Surrogate Mothers Online is to provide information and
  support to individuals who are interested in pursuing a surrogacy or
  egg and/or sperm donor arrangement. This site is created and main-
  tained through the voluntary contributions of dedicated surrogate
  mothers, egg donors, and parents via surrogacy who want to provide
  support and information to those interested in surrogacy. The site is
  not associated with any professionals in the field of surrogacy, adoption, egg donation, or sperm donation.

BabyCenter LLC
BabyCenter is the world's partner in parenting. The number one pregnancy and parenting digital destination, BabyCenter reaches more
  than forty-five million moms and dads monthly in ten languages
  and thirteen markets, from Canada to the Middle East.

The Bump
The Bump aims to connect new parents and parents-to-be. It also offers
  them personalized advice using a wide variety of user-generated con-
  tent and up-to-date community features. This includes blogs, local
  deals, checklists, personal profiles, photo galleries, topic-based message boards, and more.

Made in the USA
Monee, IL
29 December 2021

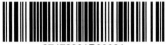